GREEN & LEAN: Get Rid of the Toxins That Make You Sick with Vegan Diet

(Eat Healthier, Lose Fat, And Be Happy)

BRIAN GREEN

This book is solely for information and educational purposes and is not medical advice. Please consult a medical or health professional before you begin any exercise, nutrition, or supplementation program or if you have questions about your health.

There may be risks associated with participating in activities or using product mentioned in this book for people in poor health or with pre-existing physical or mental health conditions.

Because these risks exist, you should not use such products or participate in such activities if you are in poor health or have a pre-existing mental or physical health conditions. If you choose to participate in these risks, you do so of your own free will and accord knowingly and voluntarily, assuming all risks associated with such activities.

Specific results mentioned in this book should be considered extraordinary and there are no "typical" results. As individuals differ, then results will differ.

TABLE OF CONTENTS

Book Description

Have you been thinking about making the vegan switch? Recently, as awareness among the general public increases a lot of people have been considering taking up veganism as their lifestyle. It's understandable that it doesn't seem to be an easy transition after having meat like chicken, fish, and beef for dinner and eggs and milk for breakfast every day of your life for the past several years. How can one give it all up so easily, and start new? Well, this book gives you all the motivation, all the right reasons and also that one last push that you're looking for to make the final decision to go vegan.

This easy-to-understand book is extremely detailed with the right sort of information that you needed to know to start veganism. It takes you into the past, telling you in detail the history, the ideology and the birth of the terminology of veganism. It fully explains the vegan diet, what it's about, its nutritional status, the foods it offers and the replacement to your meat and dairy products. It outlines a great variety of vegan recipes for you to start with and the best plant-based diets that can help you make the transition easily by slowly lowering your meat and dairy intake. It also has an entire chapter dedicated to the health, physical and other benefits that veganism has to offer along with another chapter that brings for you extreme motivation with the help of success stories. Since it's not that easy to be able understand how to go about the vegan diet when you are on your own, this book will also give you guidance with the help of tips for starters and new vegans.

Finally, and probably most importantly, the book sheds light on to a great and grave concern that our public is unaware of. This book goes into detail regarding the meat industry, its hidden agendas, its bad quality meat and horrendous treatment of animals. Going vegan, it is necessary for you to know the background and philosophy that veganism is based on so you should also know why you need to stand up against the meat industry and stop consuming what they give the public. This book reveals the truth that you and every citizen deserve to know! At the end of this book, you will be convinced that veganism is the right way of life, and you will be amazed how much there is to it. This book promises to leave out nothing that you need to and most importantly deserve to know.

INTRODUCTION

In the past couple of years, the term 'Vegan' has become mainstream and is increasingly becoming popular. This is attributed to increased awareness and a larger number of people switching to vegan diet all over the world. Veganism is a concept that was developed several years ago and has progressed in many ways to this date. Starting simply from the vegetarians of Greece and India, the concept was further established to introduce veganism and then even ethical veganism that further established the vegan philosophy.

Many people think of Veganism as a moral obligation towards animals; a responsibility towards animals to protect them and promote their basic rights of survival. However, there is much more to veganism. It has numerous health benefits that meat producing companies tend to suppress. Hidden agendas to make money by the meat producers have led to a lack of awareness regarding the health benefits of veganism and health risks of meat consumption. It is a matter of great and genuine concern that is generally overlooked by the society and conveniently ignored by the government. It is necessary for someone to highlight this genuine concern in today's world so that people are more aware of where they are headed and what their bodies are getting into. Somebody must unveil the true colors of the meat industry that is comfortably taking over.

Now veganism is not just about refraining from eating animal related foods and products but also about not using animal related products, whether they are cosmetics or clothing etc. The concept continues to grow and spread as many people bother to research and adapt veganism not just as their new diet but entirely as a new lifestyle. Vegan diet has made its way into separate sections on restaurant menus, in grocery products and even cosmetic items. Its recent popularity has led many people into finding out and researching on the topic so let us also find out what Veganism is, and everything it's about!

CHAPTER 1 –VEGANISM

WHO/WHAT IS A VEGAN?

Consider Vegans as one step ahead of vegetarians. You know that vegetarians are those people that do not consume meat (fish, cow, goat, chicken etc.) right? So Vegans, in addition to being vegetarians do not consume or use animal products such as eggs, honey, milk, other dairy products, leather, fur, wool, silk etc. Vegans follow a belief, and philosophy of refraining from the exploitation of animals in any way at all.

So basically, vegans make a statement against the exploitation of animals by boycotting their use in anything. But there are categories of vegans and clear distinctions can be established between them. Vegans can be broadly divided into three main types:

- Dietary Vegans
- Ethical Vegans
- Environmental Vegans

As the name suggests, dietary vegans refrain from consumption of meat, poultry and dairy products. But Ethical Vegans is a term applied to those vegans that not only abstain from meat consumption but also extend the vegan philosophy into other aspects of their life in which they do not make use of anything associated to animals. And finally, environmental vegans are those people that in addition to all of this, also oppose the idea of harvesting and industrial farming of animals claiming it is damaging for the environment and is unsustainable.

WHY VEGANISM?

Why people choose veganism as their diet or lifestyle is a common question. People choose to be vegan for various reasons, but mostly for health, ethical and environmental reasons.

HEALTH

Some people choose veganism for the purpose of a healthier diet and lifestyle. It is believed that once the dairy cows and egg-laying chickens become old and are no longer productive, they are sold as meat. And also, since male calves do not produce any milk, they are raised for veal and other products. So many people want to avoid these meats because of the health risks and conditions that are associated with their production. Moreover, studies have shown that the consumption of animal fats and proteins can raise your chances of developing diabetes, rheumatoid arthritis, heart diseases, cancer, hypertension, and other illnesses and diseases. Vegans also argue that the content of fat and protein in a cow's milk is very different from human milk which means that humans were not meant to consume cow's milk at all.

ANIMAL RIGHTS

Other people choose the vegan lifestyle to establish a more caring and humane attitude towards animals and promote it all over the world. They just believe they have a responsibility towards the protection of animals and their rights and do their best without being judgmental of those that do not think the same.

Some vegans believe that animals have the absolute right to live freely without the interference of humans in anything at all. Another part of this belief is that many commercially raised chickens and cows are slaughtered when they are old and unproductive. Vegans say that veganism is a cruelty-free lifestyle that follows the philosophy that animals are not ours to use, and we should not exploit them and promote their killing for our selfish benefits.

ENVIRONMENT

Then there are the third kinds of vegans that are more of tree huggers than animal lovers. Their concern is the environment. They feel that livestock farming has a damaging effect on the earth. Many vegans believe that food production through farming animals is an inefficient style of production because it uses excessive land, fertilizers, water and other resources that could be used for feeding humans instead.

Environmental vegans are of the opinion that livestock farms enhance topsoil erosion, which lowers the productivity of soil for the cultivation of crops. They also feel that a considerable amount of animal waste from factory farms pollutes the groundwater and rivers. If everyone became vegans and stopped livestock farming and production, then more people could be fed on existing land on a global scale.

CHAPTER 2 – NEW VEGAN? THINGS YOU SHOULD KNOW

TIPS FOR STARTERS

YOU DON'T HAVE TO MAKE THE SWITCH AT ONCE

Nobody expects you to become a vegan all of a sudden. Becoming one takes time and a lot of effort. A good way to start is by making your diet more plant based while also slowly reducing animal products particularly the ones that are processed and non-organic. Slowly and gradually switching to the vegan diet will help you stay motivated and wouldn't scare you away.

BE PREPARED TO READ FOOD LABELS

Becoming a vegan most certainly means that you'll have to put in the extra effort of checking the food labels for specific ingredients you intend to avoid. In today's world, most processed items that look completely non-vegan on the first sight tend to have some form of animal ingredient making it unsuitable for a vegan diet. A good example would be whey and casein, two by products of milk, which you'll find in a lot of granolas, breads and cereal bars. Similarly, ingredients like gelatin and tallow, found in a lot of candy products are derived from meat. You'll be surprised to know that Natural Red 4 (a.k.a. carmine, cochineal, or cochineal extract), a common food coloring, is made from dried bodies of female beetles. Are you sufficiently confused now? The Vegetarian Resource Group's list of most commonly used food ingredients is a good resource to start with.

YOU MAY FEEL HAPPIER

While becoming a vegan will not only make animals happier, it'll be great for you too. Here's why: Animal diet contains more arachidonic acid, an ingredient that makes certain neurological changes in humans resulting in depression, according a study by the Nutrition Journal.

YOU WON'T HAVE TO DITCH YOUR FAVORITE RESTAURANTS

The vegan movement has slowly been gaining ground and it so happens that almost every restaurant now offers great vegan options in their menu. A rule of thumb: Whenever you order something from at a restaurant, even if it looks/sounds completely vegan, does tell the waiter about your veganism to be on the safe side because a lot of these recipes tend to use chicken stock. You can also check out vegan restaurant finder com to find you the nearest and best rated vegan restaurant.

IT DOESN'T HAVE TO COST MORE

Whenever you go out for grocery shopping, at over $3 a pound, meat tends to be one of most expensive item on your list; therefore you can easily save big once you switch to vegan. You can even grow that saving by just switching your fresh products to frozen items.

PLANTS MIGHT COVER YOUR CALCIUM NEEDS

According National Institute of Health's recommendation, an average adult between the ages of 18 and 55 needs at least 1000 mg of calcium per day, but initial research shows that vegans may need much less than that. A study by a European Journal deduced that consuming at least 525 mg of calcium in a day, a vegan's chances of bone fracture are the same as that of someone on animal diet, consuming the same amount of calcium. The technique here is to eat a diverse amount of naturally calcium rich food. A good example of these foods includes bok choy, figs, kale, soy beans, navel oranges and figs. You would also find cereals, and plant-based milks which are rich in calcium along with tofu which is made of calcium sulfate. Most of the above mentioned items are also rich in Vitamin D which allows for better calcium absorption.

YOUR FRIENDS AND FAMILY WILL ASK A LOT OF QUESTIONS

Most people take their dietary habits very seriously and changing the way they think or are accustomed to think can be very difficult according to plant-based dietitian Julieanna Hever, RD, host of Veria Living's What Would Julieanna Do? "The best way to minimize conflict is to emphasize that you are going vegan for your own reasons and that it seems to work for you. In other words, make it about you, so nobody feels they need to defend their choices."

YOU'LL HAVE TO FIND NEW PROTEIN SOURCES

Protein is a must have ingredient in every meal, according to vegan dietitian Valerie Rosser, RD. They are the most important part of any organism and once broken down into amino acids, they are responsible for cellular growth and healing. According to the recommendation of the Institute of Medicine, an average adult needs to consume a minimum of 0.8 grams for every kilogram of body mass which makes it around 36 grams for a 100 pound man. According to Rosser, the best sources for vegetarian protein include seitan, lentils, natural soy, quinoa and beans.

YOU SHOULDN'T REPLACE ANIMAL PRODUCTS WITH JUNK

The most important thing to note is that becoming a vegetarian will not magically make you a healthier person. This is why it's very important not to switch to packaged food or processed breads and pasta. These items will virtually make your vegan switch a failure. Rosser said: "It's not a good idea to trade in animal products, which contain protein, vitamins, and minerals, for processed foods that provide little nutritional value other than calories." This results in a bad mood along with obesity.

CHAPTER 3 – THE VEGAN HISTORY

HOW IT BEGAN

Veganism itself is only an extension of the vegetarian concept that can be traced back to Ancient Greece and India. Vegetarianism was practiced long before it was given its name and the term only came into use in the 19th century. It was given to those people that avoided meat. Those vegetarians that even avoided eggs and dairy were attributed as total or strict vegetarians. At this point, the term vegan had no existence.

In the 19th century, numerous attempts were made in order to establish strict-vegetarian communities. These included the Temple School in Boston, Massachusetts opened by Amos Bronson Alcott in 1834. Ten years later in 1844, he also founded Fruitland's in Harvard, Massachusetts which was very short-lived. This community was against the use of animals for any purpose, even farming. This was followed by the formation of the Alcott House in Ham, Surrey in 1838 by James Pierrepont which was a community that followed strict-vegetarian diet. Then in 1847, the British Vegetarian Society was formed with the help of members of Alcott House. They held their first meeting in Ramsgate that year.

With time the concept started to progress and further discussions regarding the moral aspect of the diet led to the establishment of abstaining from animal use completely. The idea started spreading among other vegetarians and in 1851 an article was published in the Vegetarian Society's magazine that discussed using replacements for leather products. Then in 1886 the society published a Plea for Vegetarianism which demanded vegetarianism to be a moral imperative. This was done by Henry Salt who was the first to introduce a paradigm shift of animal welfare to animal rights. Salt's work is what influenced Mahatma Gandhi as well as his Ahimsa philosophy and this also led to a friendship between the two.

In 1910, the first vegan cookbook by Rupert H. Wheldon was published in London. It was called Rupert H. Wheldon's No Animal Food: Two Essays and 100 Recipes. Between the years 1909 and 1912, there was strong correspondence among the members of the Vegetarian Society regarding the ethical side of using dairy and eggs. The society's journal in 1923 stated that the "ideal position for vegetarians is abstinence from animal products." Then, finally in November 1931 Gandhi addressed the society in London in a speech which is called "The Moral Basis of Vegetarianism." He argued that the meat-free diet should be promoted as a moral issue and not just as a benefit to human health.

VEGAN – THE TERM

Leslie Cross, a member of the Leicester Vegetarian Society showed concern in the society's newsletter of July 1943 regarding the fact that vegetarians were still having cows' milk. Then in August of 1944, Donald Watson and other members of the Vegetarian Society requested for a section in the magazine for non-dairy vegetarianism. When this request was not met, he started his own newsletter that was published quarterly. This was funded by thirty readers that agreed with him.

So the first newsletter by Watson was issued in November 1944 by the name of Vegan News. That's the first time the term Vegan was used. He said that the word meant "the beginning and end of vegetarian." Other names were also suggested by readers. These included names like neo-vegetarian, allvega, vitan, dairyban, benevore, beaumangeur and sanivores. But Watson turned them all down and stuck with Vegan. This followed the formation of the new Vegan Society that held its first meeting at the Attic Club, High Holborn in London on the 15th of December in 1945. And since then World Vegan Day is held every 1st November.

Soon after this two vegan books appeared, one of which was by the Leicester Vegetarain Society. This was called Vegetarian Recipes without Dairy Produce by Margaret B. Rawls. The other book came in 1946 which was published by the Vegan Society called the Vegan Recipes by Fay K. Henderson. The definition of veganism was broadened in 1951 and became "the doctrine that man should live without exploiting animals." The society not only broadened the definition but also pledged to end animal use for anything whether it was food, hunting, work, or commodities. To further promote veganism and to make alternatives for dairy easily available, Leslie Cross founded the Plant milk Society in 1956 that explored soy milk production on a commercial scale and in 1965, Plamil Foods started the production of the first soy milks in the West. And finally in 1962, the word vegan was independently published in the Oxford Illustrated Dictionary defining vegan as "a vegetarian who eats no butter, eggs, cheese or milk."

The first vegan society of the United States came much later and was not found until 1948 by Catherine T. Nimmo of Oceano and Rubin Abramowitz of Los Angeles. Nimmo originally belonged to the Netherlands and had been a vegan since 1931. She had even been distributing the newsletter published by the Vegan Society of England actively. The next vegan society formed in the United States was by H. Jay Dinshah in 1957 that had read Watson's literature and even visited a slaughterhouse. This led him to give up all animal products and food and then on 8th February he founded the American Vegan Society in Malaga, New Jersey. He related the concept of veganism to the concept of ahimsa. The word ahimsa means "non-harming." Based on this Sanskrit word, the American Vegan Society named its magazine Ahimsa as well.

Chapter 4 – Vegan Diet

HOW DOES THE VEGAN DIET WORK?

So since being vegan means giving up all animal products including dairy and eggs, it also means taking up vegetables, fruits, leafy greens, legumes, seeds, nuts and whole grains. Veganism means lentils and veggies are your new best friends for life, and you must forget about lard, margarine and anything with gelatin.

You might feel like you're extremely limited in the variety of food you can have, but that's not true. There is still so much to choose from, and still so much you can do with your food. You can shape your diet in several ways and how you shape it is also entirely up to you. There's a great variety of delicious recipes available and you can always mix and match! And one more fun thing is that you don't have to entirely give up on dessert. You can have baked goods that don't contain eggs, butter or albumin for example cupcakes and cobbler.

If you're new to vegan diet, then make it easier for yourself by starting with a couple of meat-free dishes that you can prepare each week, and then slowly you can make more substitutions. If you also plan to lose weight, then you need to follow an exercise routine also and eat lesser calories.

VEGAN FOODS

If you're a vegan you'll have to depend on grains, seeds, beans, fruits, mushrooms and nuts for food. Common sources of plant proteins include meat analogues that are based on soybeans which is tofu, or wheat-based gluten. These are mostly in the form of vegetarian sausage, veggie burger and mince.

SOY

Since soybeans contain all the essential amino acids that humans need, they are a complete protein and can be depended upon entirely for protein consumption. This makes the entire soybean based dishes the ideal staple of vegan diets. Mostly soybeans are consumed as soy milk and tofu. Tofu is soymilk combined with a coagulant and comes in a range of textures from soft/silken for salad dressings, shakes and desserts to firm, medium firm and extra firm for stir-fries and stews. The texture of tofu depends on the water content. Apart from tofu and soymilk, soy can also be consumed in the form of texturized vegetable protein and tempeh.

PLANT MILK

Vegan diet dismissed the use of cows' or goats' milk. So instead, plant creams and milks are used in their place. These are:

- Soy milk
- Grain milks (oat or rice milk)
- Almond milk
- Coconut milk
- Hemp milk

One cup of cows' milk provides 8g of protein. On the other hand, soy milk provides 7g of protein per cup i.e. 240 ml or 8 fluid ounces. However, soy milk cannot be used to replace breast milk for the young and babies who are not breast fed need an instant formula which is mostly based on cows' milk. And when it comes to almond milk, then it is slightly lower in protein, calories and carbohydrates.

CHEESE ANALOGUES

Cheese replacements or cheese analogues are made from soy again, nuts and tapioca. Common examples of vegan cheeses are Chreese, Sheese, Teese, Daiya, and Tofutti. They easily match the taste and meltability of dairy cheese. Another common substitute for cheese in vegan recipes is nutritional yeast.You can even make cheese substitutes at home with the help of recipes from books such as the Nutritional Yeast Cookbook and The Uncheese Cookbook. A recipe even uses the combination of soy yoghurt, coconut and cashews for vegan brie. Vegan margarine such as Earth Balance can even substitute butter.

Nutrients

A matter of great concern for most people switching to vegan diet is the nutrition. Many people feel that a vegan diet will deprive them of sufficient essential nutrients and elements. This is a genuine worry that has been addressed by nutritionists all over the world and does not remain much of a problem. Fortified products and workable alternatives and replacements have been found for the convenience of vegans. Following a vegan diet strictly and getting all nutrients is not a problem anymore. Just make sure that you are aware of what your body receives because you are responsible for it, and remember to incorporate all the necessary elements in your diet. It's not that hard to be a vegan if you know what you're doing.

Before we go into detail with each nutrition you should know that vegan diets are generally richer in dietary fiber, folic acid, magnesium, vitamin E, phytochemicals and iron. On the other hand, they lack calories, cholesterol, saturated fats, vitamin D, calcium, zinc, vitamin B12, and long-chain omega-3 fatty acids. Since cleaned and uncontaminated plants do not contain vitamin B12 and may lead to deficiency if they are the only consumed foods, then it is suggested by all researchers that vegans should eat B12-fortified foods or if not, then take B12 supplements. Here is a detailed discussion on each nutrient your body needs and its relation to vegan die so that you don't have to worry about whether a vegan diet will treat your body well or not.

PROTEIN:

A vegan can easily meet protein requirements as long as his calorie intake is sufficient. You don't have to make a strict protein plan, because all you need to do is eat a varied diet. Protein is found in almost all foods so it doesn't really pose as problematic. The only foods lacking protein are alcohol, sugars and fats while all others contain some amount. For vegans, the following sources are the most suitable: tofu, chickpeas, rice, soy milk, lentils, peas, whole wheat bread, almonds, peanut butter, broccoli and spinach.

Amino acids are the building blocks of proteins. Our body requires the intake of essential amino acids, so it is important for vegans to make sure that they consume those. The combinations that contain high quantities of all the essential amino acids are beans with rice, beans with corns, and whole-wheat pita with hummus.

HERE IS A SAMPLE MENU TO MEET THE PROTEIN REQUIREMENTS IN A DAY:

- **Breakfast**

  Oatmeal (1 cup) – 6 grams

  Soy Milk (1 cup) – 7 grams

  1 Bagel (medium) – 10 grams = 23 grams

- **Lunch**

  Whole Wheat Bread (2 slices) – 7 grams

  Vegetarian Baked Beans (1 cup) – 12 grams = 19 grams

- **Dinner**

  Tofu (5 oz) – 12 grams

  Cooked Broccoli (1 cup) – 4 grams

  Almonds (2 tablespoons) – 4 grams

  Cooked Brown Rice (1 cup) – 5 grams = 25 grams

- **Snack**

  Peanut Butter (2 tablespoons) – 8 grams

  6 Crackers – 2 grams = 10 grams

TOTAL: 23+19+25+8=77 grams

The protein recommendation for a male Vegan is 63 grams, hence a diet menu such as above will suffice and give your body the right amount of proteins you need, with a full stomach.

FATS:

Generally, vegan diets are cholesterol free and are low in saturated fat. So naturally, this reduces the risk of chronic diseases of the heart and cancer. You can consume some high-fat foods but in very small amounts such as margarine, oils, seed butters, nut butters, nuts, coconut and avocado.

The government's recommendation of fat is between 20 to 35% of your daily calories. You can stay within this range if you make smart and healthful choices. As a vegan, you'll be consuming a very low quantity of fat and the fats you do get will be healthy and unsaturated kinds of fat such as those in nuts, cold-pressed oils and avocado.

VITAMIN B-12:

Vitamin B12 requirement is very low but it is highly essential for the nerve and blood cells of the body and helps to make DNA. It is also needed for normal nerve function and even cell division. However, it occurs naturally solely in animal foods so vegans have to stock up on several B-12 supplements and B-12 fortified foods. Mostly vegans are unable to obtain their B-12 from a plant-based diet so nutritionists have agreed and even stressed upon B-12 supplements for vegans. Deficiencies of Vitamin B-12 can cause several health conditions such as nerve damage, and megaloblastic anemia and can lead to problems such as weakness, tiredness, weight loss, constipation, loss of appetite and even depression.

Vegans can obtain Vitamin B-12 from non-animal sources such as Red Star nutritional yeast T6635 (Vegetarian Support Formula). You can also find numerous foods that are fortified with B-12 but always read the labels carefully before buying. You can also get your Vitamin B-12 from fortified soy milk, and supplements that do not contain animal products. Adults should aim for 2.4 micrograms of B12 because it is required for proper cell metabolism.

WHERE DOES B-12 COME FROM?

B12 is produced by microorganisms and does not directly come from plants or animals. Microorganisms such as fungi, bacteria and algae are the real makers of B12. How we get this B12 is by eating herbivorous animals that have obtained B12 from bacteria in their rumens by absorption or ingestion of their own cecotrope feces. Plants we consume that are not properly washed or contaminated water contain B12 producing bacteria. B12 that is produced in our own digestive tract is mostly expelled and we hardly retain any of our own. So evidently, increased hygiene seen particularly in the western world and developed countries is the reason for the lack of B12 in their plants. So they are left with fortified soy milk or cereal as their only choices for B12 sources.

CALCIUM:

Calcium is a crucial element of our diet because it is needed by the body to maintain bone health, vascular contraction, vasodilation, muscle function, nerve transmission, hormonal secretions and intracellular signaling. 99% of the calcium in our body is stored in our bones and teeth.

For vegans, it is recommended that they eat three servings in a day of high-calcium food for example fortified tofu, almonds, hazelnuts, or soy milk. They should even take supplements. It is found in dark green vegetables, tofu that has been made with calcium sulfate, calcium-fortified orange juice, and other vegan foods. Calcium from plants can be found in turnips, cabbage such as Chinese cabbage, broccoli and kale. Spinach however is a poor plant source of calcium. Calcium can also be found in whole-wheat bread and even grains have a small amount. Usually, vegans don't find it difficult to meet the critical need of calcium.

According to the EPIC-Oxford study, vegans have a higher risk of bone fractures in comparison to meat eaters and even vegetarians. This is probably because of their lower dietary calcium intake. As a vegan, you should consider it as your responsibility to make sure that you are getting enough. The advised calcium intake for average adults 19-50 years of age is 1000 mgs/day.

Note: Calcium absorption needs Vitamin D, so vegans have to make sure they have sufficient vitamin D as well which is discussed later. Also, oxalic acid is found in chards, rhubarb, beet greens and spinach. It binds with the calcium present in those foods which reduces its absorption. This is why these foods are not your best sources of calcium and should not be considered if you're trying to increase calcium intake. However, in other green veggies calcium is well absorbed and dietary fiber has almost no effect on calcium absorption.

For you to have a better idea of your calcium intake here are calcium content values of some selected vegan foods for you to choose from:

HERE ARE SAMPLE MENUS FOR MEALS THAT PROVIDE MORE THAN 1000 MGS OF CALCIUM IN A DAY:

Food	Amount	Calcium (mg)
Cooked broccoli	1 cup	62
Plain commercial soy yogurt	6 ounce	300
Calcium-fortified, plain and commercial soy or rice milk	8 ounces	200-300
Cooked okra	1 cup	135
Tempeh	1 cup	184
Cooked turnip greens	1 cup	249
Processed Tofu - with calcium sulfate	4 ounces	200-420
Processed Tofu- with nigari	4 ounces	130-400
Cooked kale	1 cup	179
Cooked mustard greens	1 cup	152
Tahini	2 tbsps.	128
Cooked navy beans	1 cup	126
Cooked Bok choy	1 cup	158
Almond butter	2 tbsps.	111
Cooked soybeans	1 cup	175
Whole Almonds	1/4 cup	94
Other calcium-fortifiedplant milks	8 ounces	300-500
Calcium-fortified orange juice	8 ounces	350
Cooked collard greens	1 cup	357
Blackstrap molasses	2 tbsps.	400

CALCIUM (MG)
BREAKFAST:

1 cup Calcium-Fortified Soy Milk   300

1 serving Cindy's Light and Fluffy Pancakes 195

LUNCH:

6 Dried Figs   82

1 serving of Hummus on Pita Bread

178

1/4 cup of Almonds 94

DINNER:

Scrambled Tofu and Bok Choy over Brown Rice 190

Green Salad and Tangerine Dressing   30

Chocolate Pudding 92

TOTAL   1161

BREAKFAST:

2 tablespoons of Almond Butter   111

1 Toasted medium Bagel with   93

1 serving Tropical Fruit Smoothie 102

LUNCH:

1 serving of Creamed Spinach   121

1 serving of Mini Pizzas   235

DINNER:

1 cup of Steamed Broccoli	62
1 serving of Chocolate Pudding	92
1 serving of Lemon Rice Soup	82
1 serving of Tofu Squash Burgers	135
TOTAL	1033

IRON:

There isn't much difference in the iron content of vegan diet and animal-based diets. In fact, vegan diets contain more iron than vegetarian diets because dairy products hardly have any iron in them anyway. However, concerns arise related to the bioavailability of iron when it is taken from plant sources as researchers say that it is only 5-15% from plants and 18% from non-vegetarian iron sources. The incidence of iron deficiency anemia is not seen more in vegans than in non-vegetarians but since the bioavailability is lower supplements should be used but only upon consultation with a physician because excessive iron can be toxic for the body.

Good sources of iron for vegans include dark leafy vegetables and dried beans. For better absorption of Iron, consume foods containing vitamin C along with foods containing iron and avoid having anything that would stop absorption such as tannin in tea. Your sources of vitamin C can be orange juice, or cauliflower consumed with iron sources such as black beans or tofu. Avoid herbal teas, coffees and spices containing tannins as they lower the absorption of iron. Vegetarian Resource Group suggests that high-iron foods that are good for vegans are lentils, tofu, kidney beans, quinoa, chickpeas, and black-strap molasses.

Some other sources of iron are: black-eyed peas, tempeh, prune juice, Swiss chard, beet greens, peas, tahini, raisins, watermelon and millet.

For the sake of your information, and so that you have an accurate idea of how much iron you are consuming here is a list of the iron contents of some selected common iron containing foods:

1 CUP OF EACH:
- Cooked lentils 6.6 mgs
- Cooked kidney beans 5.2 mgs
- Cooked soybeans 8.8 mgs
- Cooked chickpeas 4.7 mgs
- Cooked Swiss chad 4.0 mgs
- Cooked Lima beans 4.5 mgs

VITAMIN D:

Vitamin D is needed by our body for various functions such as calcium absorption, bone growth and mineralization process of bone. Deficiency of vitamin D can cause bones to become fragile, brittle and thin. It works with calcium to protect us from osteoporosis. It is produced inside our body when sun rays containing UV radiation hit our skin.

Vegan diet is almost devoid of any vitamin D and hardly any plant sources provide vitamin D. The only source of vitamin D for vegans is through exposure to sunlight or through fortified foods. For sufficient Vitamin D you need at least 10-15 minutes of exposure to the sun on your hands and face thrice a week so that it can be produced. Apart from the sun, your food sources are only vitamin D-fortified soy and rice milk. If your exposure to the sun is limited, then you need to take additional supplements to make sure you fulfill your body's critical vitamin D requirement.

There are two forms of Vitamin D: Colecalciferol (D3) and Ergocalciferol (D2). Colecalciferol is the form of vitamin D that is synthesized in the skin from sun exposure or comes from animal products. On the other hand, Ergocalciferol comes from ergosterol in yeast so is more favorable for Vegans. There are still some conflicting studies that suggest that the two forms may or not be bioequivalent. However, according to the Nutritional Board of the National Academy of Science both of them function as prohormones and their differences do not affect metabolism. They show identical responses in the body.

Looking solely at vitamin D related to sun exposure, then whether the sunlight is sufficient or not depends on the time of the day and the season. It also depends on the skin melanin content and if there is any sunscreen covering the skin. It has been suggested by the National Institutes of Health, that most people can get enough vitamin D from the sun spring, fall and obviously summer, even those that are living in the far north. According to them, only a 5-30 minute exposure to the sun from 10 in the morning to 3 in the afternoon twice in a week is good enough.

OMEGA 3 FATTY ACIDS AND IODINE:
Omega-3 fatty acids such asAlpha-linolenic acids (ALA) are found in nuts, leafy green vegetables, vegetable oils like canola and flaxseed oil, tofu, soybeans and walnuts. Vegans should include these good sources of ALA in their diets. It is advised that vegans take a quarter of a teaspoon of flaxseed oil/linseed oil every day, and take oils with less quantities of omega-6 fatty acids like avocado, peanut or olive oil.

In places and countries where the salt is not typically iodized, vegans will probably have to take Iodine supplementation also. Iodine supplements may even is necessary if salt is iodized at low levels or if dairy products are depended upon for iodine due to lack of availability in the soil. Iodine is available in most multivitamins for vegans and can also be found in seaweeds like kelp.

REPLACEMENT OF DAIRY PRODUCTS AND EGGS
The concept of Veganism is based against the consumption of eggs and dairy products as they believe that the production of eggs and dairy has a lot to do with animal suffering and premature death. So this clearly demands and emphasized the necessity of substitutions and appropriate replacements for these foods as they are a critical need of the human body. A lot of the food we eat that is not dairy or eggs contain dairy and eggs so this requires the production of egg-free vegan forms of the same products. For

example, egg-free/vegan mayonnaise brands can be found such as Veganaise, Miso Mayo, Nayonaise and Plamil's Egg-Free Mayo.

Egg is not only an ingredient in several food products but is also used in numerous recipes for the purpose of thickening or binding because the protein found in egg thickens when heated and binds ingredients together. So what do vegans do when they want an egg-free product but need the same effect? Well, this effect can be achieved using ground flax seeds if you simply replace each egg in the recipe with a tablespoon of flaxseed and three tablespoons of water.

Pancakes are absolutely delicious and who can live without those? I am sure you can't either. But don't worry, just because you're vegan doesn't mean you have to give them up also! You can simply use one tablespoon of baking powder instead of the eggs. The job done is the same.

Other substitutes for eggs as binders:

- 1 small mashed banana
- 2 ounces of soft tofu mixed with other liquid ingredients
- ¼ cup of applesauce
- 2 tablespoons of arrowroot starch or cornstarch

For other dairy products, you can look into the following substitutions:

- Potato milk, soy milk, nut milk, rice milk or water
- Soured soy or rice milk to replace buttermilk (1 cup soymilk with 1 tablespoon of vinegar)
- Soy cheese (make sure it has no casein)
- Crumbled tofu to replace cottage or ricotta cheese in food such as lasagna
- Non-dairy cream cheese is also available

CHAPTER 5 – RECIPES

Being a vegan means a lot of work when it comes to having food. You need to be very particular and make sure that you consume the right sort of food with all the nutrients in the sufficient amount. That takes a good amount of research and time to be certain that you get your food right. You cannot depend on others for what you consume anymore if you have made the vegan switch. So for your convenience, here are a bunch of amazing recipes that favor all your desires and nutritional needs as a vegan. These vegan recipes are not just tasty but also fulfil your nutritional requirement. If you're looking for something helps you lose weight, develop strong bones yet gain muscle then these are for you.

The following recipes are divided according to their types: soups, main dishes, deserts and any side dishes to ensure that you get everything you want and you're left satisfied without any meaty guilt!

SOUPS

VEGAN RED LENTIL SOUP
INGREDIENTS
- Peanut oil – 1 tablespoon
- Fresh minced ginger root – 1 tablespoon
- Chopped small onion - 1
- Chopped clove garlic - 1
- Dry red lentils – 1 cup
- Coconut milk – ½ can/14 ounces
- Tomato paste – 2 tablespoons
- Fenugreek seeds – 1 pinch
- Finely chopped fresh cilantro – 1/3 cup
- Cayenne pepper – 1 pinch
- Salt and pepper – add to taste

- Butternut squash (peeled, seeded, and cubed) – 1 cup
- Curry powder – 1 teaspoon
- Ground nutmeg – 1 pinch
- Water – 2 cups

DIRECTIONS

- Using only medium heat, heat the oil in a large pot and cook the garlic, onion, fenugreek, and ginger until the onion becomes tender.
- Then add the squash, cilantro and lentils into the pot and mix. Also add the coconut milk, water, tomato paste and stir them in.
- Finally season using the cayenne pepper, curry powder, salt, pepper and nutmeg.
- Allow it to come to a boil, and then lower the heat. Simmer for 30 minutes or until the squash and lentils become tender. There, you've already learnt how to prepare one vegan soup. What a perfect start!

VEGAN HOT AND SOUR SOUP
INGREDIENTS
- Dried wood ear mushrooms – 1 ounce
- Rice vinegar – 5 tablespoons
- Sesame oil – ½ tablespoon
- Dried shiitake mushrooms - 4
- Soy sauce – 3 tablespoons
- Bamboo fungus – 1/3 ounce
- Vegetable broth – 1 quart
- Chili oil – ½ tablespoon
- Ground black pepper – ½ teaspoon
- Dried tiger lily buds - 12
- Crushed red pepper flakes – ¼ teaspoon
- Cornstarch – ¼ cup
- Hot water – 2 cups

- Ground white pepper – ¾ teaspoon
- Chinese dried mushrooms – 1 cup
- Firm tofu – 8 ounce/1 container (cut into ¼ inch strips)
- Sliced green onion – 1

DIRECTIONS

- Place the lily buds, wood mushrooms and shiitake mushrooms in one small bowl with 1.5 cups of hot water. Let it soak for 20 minutes until rehydrated and then drain. Then, trim the stems from all the mushrooms and cut them into thin strips. And chop the lily buds in equal halves.
- Using another small bowl containing ¼ cup of slightly salted hot water, soak bamboo fungus for 20 minutes. Again, until rehydrated. Then drain and mince.
- Then, in a third bowl add rice vinegar, soy sauce and 1 tablespoon of cornstarch and blend these together. Then add ½ of the tofu strips into the mix.
- Add the reserved mushroom and lily bud liquid from the first bowl into a medium saucepan and mix it with the vegetable broth. Let it boil and then stir in your shiitake and wood mushroom and lily bud. Lower the heat and simmer for 5 minutes. And then season with black, red and white pepper.
- Then mix the remaining cornstarch and water in a small bowl. Stir them into the broth mixture and continue until you think it has thickened.
- Add the soy sauce and remaining tofu strips into the saucepan, and allow it to boil again. Stir in the bamboo fungus, sesame oil and the chili oil. Finally, garnish with the green onion and its ready to be served!

MAIN DISHES

VEGAN LASAGNA
INGREDIENTS
- Olive oil – 2 tablespoons
- Minced garlic – 3 tablespoons
- Chopped onion – 1 ½ cups

- Lasagna noodles – 1 package (16 ounce)
- Stewed tomatoes – 4 cans (14.5 ounce)
- Chopped fresh basil – ½ cup
- Minced garlic – 2 tablespoons
- Frozen chopped spinach, thawed and drained – 3 packages (10 ounce)
- Tomato paste – 1/3 cup
- Salt – 1 teaspoon
- Chopped fresh basil – ¼ cup
- Chopped parsley – ½ cup
- Firm tofu – 2 pounds
- Ground black pepper – 1 teaspoon
- Chopped parsley – ¼ cup
- Ground black pepper – add to taste
- Salt – ½ teaspoon

DIRECTIONS

- Start by making the sauce. Use a heavy, large saucepan to heat olive oil over medium heat. Then add onions into the saucepan and saute them until soft. This should take about 5 minutes. Then add the garlic and cook for a further 5 more minutes.
- Then add your tomatoes, the tomato paste, parsley and basil into the saucepan as well and stir well. Reduce the heat and allow the sauce to simmer covered for an hour. Then add your salt and pepper.
- As the sauce cooks, boil a large kettle of salted water. Boil the lasagna noodles for 9 minutes, drain the water and then rinse.
- Preheat your oven – 200 degrees C/ 400 degrees F
- Take a large bowl and put the tofu blocks in it. Then add basil, parsley and garlic. Also add salt and pepper and then mix all the ingredients inside together with the help of your fingers. Squeeze the pieces of tofu well.

- Finally, assemble the lasagna. First spread the tomato sauce (only 1 cup) at the bottom of casserole pan (9x13 inches). Then arrange one layer of lasagna noodles and sprinkle the tofu mixture on top. Then add the spinach evenly over the layer of tofu and pour 1.5 cups of tomato sauce over the tofu. Add another layer of noodles. Just like before, sprinkle another 1/3 tofu mixture on top of the noodles, then add 1.5 more cups of tomato sauce and again top with a last layer of noodles above the tomato sauce. Then at the end, sprinkle the last 1/3 of the tofu mixture and spread your remaining tomato sauce on the top.
- Foil up your lasagna to cover it and then allow it to bake for 30 minutes.

VEGAN FAJITA
INGREDIENTS

- Olive oil - ¼ cup
- Chili powder – 1 teaspoon
- Red wine vinegar – ¼ cup
- Garlic salt – add to taste
- Salt and pepper– add to taste
- Black beans, drained – 1 can (15 ounce)
- Dried oregano – 1 teaspoon
- Whole kernel corn, drained – 1 can (8.75 ounce)
- Small zucchini, julienned – 2
- White sugar – 1 teaspoon
- Large onion, sliced - 1
- Medium small yellow squash, julienned - 2
- Olive oil – 2 tablespoons
- Green bell pepper– 1 (cut into thin strips)
- Red bell pepper – 1 (cut into thin strips)

DIRECTIONS

- Take a large bowl and mix olive oil, chili powder, vinegar, garlic salt, oregano, sugar, salt and pepper. Add zucchini, onion, green and red pepper, and yellow squash. Keep the vegetables in the refrigerator for 30 minutes at least but not for more than 24 hours for marination.
- Use a large skillet to heat oil over medium-high heat. After draining, add the vegetables and saute them until they're soft. This will take 10-15 minutes. Then stir the corn and beans, and increase the heat for 5 minutes to make sure the vegetables turn brown.

VEGAN BREAKFAST

VEGAN CREPES
INGREDIENTS

- Soy milk – ½ cup
- Turbinado sugar – 1 tablespoon
- Melted soy margarine – ¼ cup
- Unbleached all-purpose flour – 1 cup
- Water – ½ cup
- Salt – ¼ teaspoon
- Maple syrup – 2 tablespoons

DIRECTIONS

- Use a large mixing bowl to combine water, soy milk, sugar, flour, salt, syrup and ¼ cup margarine. Then cover the bowl and chill the combination for 2 hours.
- With the help of some soy margarine, grease a 5-6 inch skillet lightly. Then, heat the skillet until it becomes hot and pour about 3 tablespoons of the batter inside it. Then allow it to cook until it becomes golden and then flip it to cook the opposite side till it becomes golden as well.

VEGAN PANCAKES

INGREDIENTS

- Rye flour – ½ cup
- Whole wheat flour – ½ cup
- Soy flour – 1 tablespoon
- Soy milk – ½ cup
- Baking powder – 1 ½ teaspoons
- Chopped pecans – ¼ cup
- White sugar – 1 tablespoon
- Water – ½ cup
- Salt – 1/8 teaspoon
- Ground cinnamon (optional) – 1/8 teaspoon
- Vanilla extract (optional) – ½ teaspoon

DIRECTIONS

- Take a medium bowl and combine the three flours: wheat, rye, and soy. Also stir in the salt, cinnamon, baking powder and sugar. Then make a well in the center and pour the water, vanilla and soy milk inside. Once done, mix the combination until you're sure that the dry ingredients have been absorbed and then add the pecans. Stir them in.
- Heat up a griddle iron or a large skillet over medium heat and coat with cooking spray. Then pour 1/3 cup of batter on its hot surface and spread the batter to ¼ inch in thickness. Let it cook until bubble start to appear on the surface. When that happens, flip and cook the other side to brown. Then you can finally serve it warm.

DESERTS

VEGAN CUPCAKES
INGREDIENTS
- All-purpose flour – 2 cups
- Baking powder – 2 teaspoons
- Apple cider vinegar – 1 tablespoon
- Baking soda – ½ teaspoon
- Almond milk – 1 ½ cup
- Vanilla extract – 1 ¼ teaspoons
- White sugar – 1 cup
- Coconut oil, warmed until liquid – ½ cup
- Salt – ½ teaspoon

DIRECTIONS
- First grease two 12 cup muffin pans or you can use 18 paper baking cups. Also, preheat your oven to 175 degrees C/350 degrees F.
- Using a 2 cup measuring cup, measure the apple cider vinegar in it and then fill with almond milk to make 1 ½ cups. Leave it to stand until it curdles. This will take about 5 minutes. Then take a large bowl to combine flour, baking powder, sugar, salt and baking soda. Take a separate bowl and whisk coconut oil, vanilla and almond milk mixture together. Then mix both the ingredients i.e. the pour the wet mixture into the dry mixture and stir to blend. Once your batter is ready, spoon it out into the prepared muffin pans/baking cups making sure you distribute evenly.
- Allow the cupcakes to bake for 15-20 minutes in the preheated oven. The tops should spring back when they are slightly pressed. That means you stop baking and let the pan cool by setting it over a wire rack. Once it has cooled, arrange the cupcakes on a serving dish and frost the way you want.

VEGAN PUDDING
INGREDIENTS
- Cornstarch – 3 tablespoons
- Soy milk – 1 ½ cups
- Vanilla extract – ¼ teaspoon
- Unsweetened cocoa powder – ¼ cup
- Water – 2 tablespoons
- White sugar – ¼ cup

DIRECTIONS
- Mix the cornstarch and water to form a paste in a small bowl.
- Take a large saucepan, and stir in vanilla, soy milk, sugar, cornstarch mixture and cocoa over medium heat. Then cook the mixture in the saucepan and keep stirring until you see that the mixture is boiling. Continue cooking and keep stirring. When the mixture thickens, remove it from the heat. Then allow it to cool, and the pudding will still continue to thicken. Let it be for five minutes and then put it in the refrigerator to chill. Take out later when you think it's ready.

SIDE DISHES

VEGAN BAKED BEANS
INGREDIENTS
- Dry navy beans – 1 package (16 ounce)
- Olive oil – 2 tablespoons
- Molasses – ¼ cup
- Ground black pepper – ¼ teaspoon
- Chopped sweet onions – 2 cups
- Ground nutmeg – ¼ teaspoon
- Cider vinegar – 2 tablespoons
- Tomato sauce – 4 cans (8 ounce)
- Water – 6 cups

- Ground cinnamon – ¼ teaspoon
- Bay leaves – 3
- Clove garlic, minced – 1
- Firmly packed brown sugar – ¼ cup
- Dry mustard – 1 teaspoon

DIRECTIONS

- Take a large pot to put beans and water in and then let it boil. Lower the heat to a medium level once boiling starts and keep cooking for 1 hour. Stir every now and then and stop when you see the beans are tender. Then drain and transfer ingredients into a large casserole dish.
- Preheat oven to 150 degrees C/300 degrees F.
- Using only medium heat, heat the olive oil in a skillet. Stir in the onions and cook them until they are tender before you add the garlic. Cook the garlic as well until it turns golden brown. Then transfer the cooked onions and garlic into the casserole dish containing the beans and mix. Then pour the tomato sauce as well and stir. Finally add the molasses, brown sugar, bay leaves, mustard pepper, vinegar, nutmeg, and cinnamon. Stir.
- Cover the dish and bake for 3 ½ hours in the preheated oven. Remember to stir frequently and if need arises, you can add water if you think necessary. Then bake for another 30 minutes after removing the cover.

VEGAN SWEET POTATO STICKS
INGREDIENTS
- Olive oil – 1 tablespoon
- Sweet potatoes – 8 (sliced into quarters lengthwise)
- Paprika – ½ teaspoon

DIRECTIONS

- First preheat your oven to 200 degrees C/400 degrees F and use cooking spray or vegetable oil over your baking sheet.
- Mix oil and paprika in a large bowl and then add the potato sticks. Then use your hands to stir and coat. Once you're done coating, place it on the prepared baking sheet.
- Finally bake for 40 minutes only in the preheated oven and then remove from the oven. Let it cool down a bit because it's best eaten at room temperature.

Chapter 6 – The Best Plant-based Diets

So far you know what vegan diet is about, the nutrition it offers and you even know ten recipes that you can start with. However, it's not easy to make a sudden switch from a meat-eater to a vegan and start eating all the vegetables and fruits without a tinge of meat or eggs. To help make your switch much easier and give you a greater variety of foods you can eat, there are ready-made plant-based diets that are good for your health and heart. They are not entirely vegan or vegetarian and are not completely devoid of meat and dairy but they are a great way for you to start adopting the vegan diet. It takes time for your body to get used to the lack of meat, and your taste buds to forget meat and live without the temptation. So for this purpose, and to make your transition more comfortable this chapter gives you the best-plant based diets that you can choose from. These plant- based diets are healthy because they require minimally processed foods from plants, and use plant protein instead of animal protein; they contain a modest amount of fish, lean meat and low-fat dairy. These diets hardly use any red meat that is why they are the perfect solution to make an easier transition.

THE MEDITERRANEAN DIET
Old ways, a nonprofit food think tank in Boston worked with the Harvard School of Public Health to develop a consumer-friendly and easy Mediterranean diet pyramid that revolves around fruits, veggies, nuts, legumes, beans, whole grains, spices, herbs and olive oil. It involves the consumption of fish only around twice a week, poultry in moderate amounts and red meat and sweets only occasionally.

This diet provides you with an eating pattern but not an exactly structured diet plan so it leaves you to figure out your own Mediterranean menu, your calorie intake, and activities you want to do to stay fit.

THE FLEXITARIAN DIET
The Flexitarian Diet requires you to add five food group to your meals and your diet overall. These five groups of food are:

- The 'New meat' which is peas, seeds, nuts, lentils, tofu and beans
- Fruits and vegetables
- Dairy
- Whole grains
- Sugar and spice

The Flexitarian five week meal plan has breakfast, lunch, snacks and dinner recipes that you can follow as outlined but you can also switch and exchange recipes from different weeks according to your own preferences. This diet can be tough if you don't enjoy fruits and vegetables but it's flexible, it's delicious and is all done at home. The Flexitarian plan offers 300 calories in breakfast, 400 calories in lunch and 500 calories in dinner so it's a 3-4-5 regimen. Snacks about 150 calories each so if you have two in a day then your total calorie intake in a single day is 1500 calories.

The meals in this diet revolve around the consumption of plant proteins instead of animal proteins. For breakfast, you have cereal topped with soy milk instead of cattle milk and nuts and berries; for lunch you have a black bean soup alongside a salad and a whole-grain roll; for a snack you can have an apple with peanut butter which is delicious, and finally for dinner go for a barbeque veggie burger with sweet potato fries.

THE ORNISH DIET
This diet has been developed by a professor at the University of California, Sanfrancisco, Dean Ornish. He categorizes food into five groups as well from group 1 foods being the most healthful and group 5 being the least. The difference is just like the difference between having whole-grain bread and having biscuits or the difference between soy hot dogs and beef ones. Apart from the diet, Ornish also emphasizes on aerobic activities, flexibility and resistance training. You get to decide what you want to do and when. For better results with an ornish diet, also make time for meditation, deep breathing and yoga. This helps you manage you stress so find out a combination that works for you and do it every day. Dean Ornish also stresses on spending time with people you love and respect, and using their support because they can affect your health in the greatest of ways.

Everything that Ornish has suggested for healthy living can be applied to fight a host of common health problems such as cholesterol levels, obesity, blood pressure, type 2 diabetes, breast cancer, prostate cancer and heart diseases. If you take this up, your heart will love you!

THE TRADITIONAL ASIAN DIET

Old ways has also developed a consumer-friendly and easy Asian diet pyramid that revolves around a diet of noodles, rice, bread, corn, millet and other whole-grains taken every day. This diet is extremely filling with diverse foods and flavors. It might be hard for people who don't enjoy rice or noodles so they have other diets to choose from. The diet also needs you to have a good amount of legumes, fruits, veggies, nuts, seeds and vegetable oils. It only allows eggs, poultry and something sweet once in a week and red meat only once a month. Fish and shellfish are optional. The pyramid also requires the consumption of six glasses of water or tea every day and wine, sake and beer are only allowed in moderation. Make sure that you keep yourself physically active, and you're good.

Veggies and tubers part of the Asian diet are bean sprouts, book choy, bitter melons, bamboo shoots, carrots, leeks, eggplants, turnips, galangals, yams and sweet potatoes. Examples of fruits taken in the Asian Diet include mangoes, tangerines, rambutan, coconuts and apricots. According to Old ways, you can get your grain in the Asian diet by stressing on having rice, noodles, naan, dumplings, barley and buckwheat. Noodles could be rice noodles, or udon, somen or soba. Additionally, if you choose to have fish then you can choose from clams, octopus, eels, mussels, abalone and cockles. Finally, examples of herbs and spices you would like to put in your Asian diet are basil, masala, turmeric, mint, clove, curry leaves, amchoor and fennel.

Chapter 7 – The Benefits of Vegan Diet

Why Vegan diet is good for you is a common question with several answers! The great thing about vegan diet is that it has way too many advantages not just for you but for the environment, for people around you, for animals and for the world you live in. Just by switching to vegan and giving up eggs and meat you can do yourself the biggest favor you have ever done. Switching to a vegan diet is the best decision you will probably make in your whole life because it will bring the best of changes for you and improve your lifestyle remarkably.

The benefits of vegan diet range from health, skin, lifestyle and environment. Once you get the hang of it, you'll realize all the goodness you have achieved. It's important that you know why vegan diet is so good for you for the sake of your motivation.

There are numerous success stories in terms of weight loss or improved health by pursuing vegan diet. A great number of people have gotten rid of cardiovascular and obesity problems with the help of the consumption of fruits and vegetables only. Let's look into the details of the benefits of vegan diets so that you can understand why it's the most perfect plan for you!

HEALTH BENEFITS
Your body is the most important thing to you. More than anything you want to stay fit and healthy and stay away from diseases of the heart, kidneys, lungs and even cancers. Your health is greatly, in fact mostly affected by what you feed your body. Only you are responsible for taking care of your health and what you ingest on a daily basis. Following a vegan diet plan will make that job easier for you because it will keep you healthy in uncountable ways. You will realize that keeping healthy was never made this easy before. Here are a number of health benefits of vegan diet.

No Heart problems

Your heart is the most vital organ of your body and you must ensure that it runs and functions properly at all times. Consumption of red meats and others such poses several health risks to your cardiovascular system. In fact, they say that the best way to keep heart diseases at bay and your blood pressure and cholesterol level under control is an eating pattern light on fat and heavy on veggies and fruits. In general, consuming nuts and whole grain without eating any meat and dairy products will improve your cardiovascular health considerably. You don't have to worry about heart attacks and strokes as such because your diet is the biggest predisposing factor of such diseases and if kept in control, then you are free of any such problems.

Many studies have proven the beneficial effects of vegan diet on the heart. One such study compared 6000 vegans to 5000 meat consumers. It was a 12 year study in which researchers discovered that vegans were at a 57% lower risk of ischemic heart disease than those that had meat and the vegetarians had a 24% lower risk. The vegans did better than both the other groups because even eggs and cheese increase the risk of heart diseases. When the study ended, the results showed that the vegans had the lowest total and LDL cholesterol.

PROTECTION FROM CANCERS

Overall, vegans appear to have a greater life expectancy and lower cancer rates in comparison to other people living in the same environment and community. Vegans are generally also more concerned about their health and tend to stay away from other cancer-causing practices such as smoking or consuming alcohol. This further reduces their chances of developing cancer.

When high-fat processed red meats are cooked at high temperatures, they may give rise to cancerous compounds. The metabolism of these compounds produces risk factors for the development of cancer. It is also said that extra amounts of iron can also promote reactive free radicals to be formed and damage cells. Additionally, some researchers have even provided evidence of a direct relationship between heme iron, red meat, and high temperature cooking and cancer development.

Prostate cancer: A major study provides evidence that men with early stage prostate cancer who changed their diet and started vegan managed to control the cancer from progressing and some of them even managed to reverse the cancer process.

COLON CANCER: The risk of colon cancer is also greatly reduced by eating a diet consisting of whole grains as well as fruits and vegetables.

BREAST CANCER: Studies show that in countries with women who are not consuming as much meat and animal products are less prone to the development of breast cancer. These countries have shown a much lower rate of breast cancer than those countries where women consume large amounts of meat and animal products. The lowered incidence of breast cancer in vegans is attributed to the fact that vegans have lower levels of estrogen in their blood, longer menstrual cycles, and a later onset of menstruation as well. This results in the reduced exposure to estrogen.

PREVENTION OF DIABETES

Vegan diet successfully acts as weapon against type 2 diabetes as well. In fact, it is easier to follow than the standard diet recommended for the diabetic patients by the American Diabetic Association. Vegan and vegetarian diets are significantly helpful in the management and prevention of diabetes. A considerably lower risk of type 2 diabetes has been observed in individuals pursuing a veg diet in comparison to meat eaters. According to the original Adventist Health Study, vegetarians and vegans had almost half the risk of developing diabetes. Moreover, the study also showed a significant relationship between increased diabetes risk and red meat consumption regardless of other dietary factors, body weight and physical activity.

It is still confusing and unclear whether the reduced risk in diabetes in vegans and vegetarians is because of reduced meat intake or increased plant food (grains, legumes, nuts). But it is very clear because of several studies that there is a positive link between heme iron consumption through red meat and the risk of type 2 diabetes. There is also evidence of a positive association between taking red meat, animal proteins and processed meat and the occurrence of type 2 diabetes.

Apart from the absence of red meat in diet, there are several other aspects of vegan diet that help in prevention and management of diabetes. Following a vegan diet also means a reduced intake of saturated fat and an increased intake of whole grains, nuts, dietary fiber and legumes. This sort of a diet has demonstrated a reduced risk of diabetes as well. Moreover, the substitution of animal protein with soy and vegetable protein has also shown to reduce the risk and progress of renal diseases associated with both types of diabetes.

PREVENTION OF ARTHRITIS, KIDNEY DISEASE AND CATARACTS

It has long been considered that the elimination of dairy consumption alleviates the symptoms of arthritis, but recently newer studies have even demonstrated that a combination of vegan and gluten-free diet is extremely helpful in improving the health conditions of patients of rheumatoid arthritis. Studies show that individuals that suffer from rheumatoid arthritis will feel better with a low fat vegan or vegetarian diet after a period of fasting. The mechanism behind these improvements in the health of arthritic patients is unclear but it is somehow related to reduction in the process of inflammation. According to a review of four controlled studies each of which lasted three months, there is a clinically significant effect of such diets on arthritis.

Moreover, it has been noted that increased consumption of animal protein can produce adverse effects for those that have underlying kidney issues. According to a study of individuals with type 2 diabetes, renal function can improve by the elimination of red meat from the diet and having a low-protein diet. Similarly, in patients that have type 1 diabetes, replacement of animal protein by soy and vegetable protein has shown improved kidney function as well. Another study of individuals with type 2 diabetes and nephropathy also demonstrated that the replacement of 35% animal protein with soy protein lowered the incidence of urinary creatinine and proteinuria.

Another disease known as cataracts is also eliminated and headed off with the help of vegan diet by the intake of fruits and vegetables. Fruits that contain high amounts of antioxidants help prevent diseases like cataracts.

PHYSICAL BENEFITS

Staying healthy is one thing, and staying fit is another. In fact, the two things go hand in hand. In order to stay healthy, you need to stay fit. You can't let yourself gain too much weight or lose too much weight because both extremes lead to health related problems and conditions. So the good news is, vegan diet isn't only going to help you stay healthy, it also fulfils the fitness aspect as well. It looks after your weight, your bones and your muscles. Pursuing a vegan diet will give you physical benefits that will make you a lot more energetic, attractive and much stronger as well.

BODY MASS INDEX

Numerous studies regarding diet have shown that a diet lacking meat results in a lower BMI. A low BMI is indicative of a healthy fat and less fat. A study has demonstrated a considerable difference in the BMI between four different kinds of diet groups. The study shows that the meat eaters had the highest BMI, followed by vegetarians and fish eaters, and the lowest BMI was seen in vegans. The difference in BMI is attributed to the differences in macronutrient intake between meat eaters and vegans. There is a strong association between high protein and low fiber intake and increasing BMI.

WEIGHT LOSS

Weight loss is typically seen as a result of a smart vegan diet. The weight loss that results is healthy and reverses the conditions of obesity and over-weight individuals. This is because eating vegan rids you off the unhealthy foods that unnecessarily contribute to your weight and gives you the perfect amount of all nutrients without any excessive weight gain. An increased consumption of red meat has been associated to an increased risk of weight gain while on the other hand; foods such as whole grains and nuts are independently linked to reduced risk of weight gain and obesity.

Energy

A healthy vegan diet also leads to more energy. You will find yourself feeling a lot more energetic and less lethargic at the end of every day once you start pursuing a vegan diet strictly. This is because vegan diets are free of cholesterol-laden animal products that slow us down physically and make us feel tired every morning we try to wake up to. But since vegan diet contains all sorts of grains, fruits and legumes, they are high in complex carbohydrates that provide a great amount of energizing fuel for the body and as a result every morning you feel zapped and full of energy!

HEALTHY SKIN

This is a fascinating and popular benefit of vegan diet that many people have noticed for themselves. After following a vegan diet several people have noticed remarkable changes in their skin. This is attributed to the nuts and vegetables containing vitamins A and E as they play a huge role in healthy skin. As a result, most vegans end up in a good and healthy skin and will notice a significant reduction in the blemishes they had before.

Healthy vegan meals are loaded with vitamins C and E which are strong antioxidants that function to help reduce wrinkles, and brown spots. They also defuse the effect of skin-damaging free radicals, which automatically gives an overall youthful and fresh look to your skin. Primarily, vitamin E is found in nuts and seeds and you can help your skin simply by munching and chewing on almonds, ground flax seeds, walnuts and even sunflower seeds. If you're looking for an easy way to get your vitamin E then another option is stocking up on peanut butter and if you want a sweeter taste to your antioxidants then you can also go for a bunch of berries to meet that need. You never thought making your skin look fresher and neater was this easy before, did you?

An article recently published in the Health magazine supported the action of zinc found in beans against zits. Zinc reduces inflammation, redness and rids your skin of pimples as well. Dairy products, which are exclusively excluded from vegan diet are a contributing factor to acne so once you stop taking those, you clearly get rid of a predisposition. In fact, your vegan protein sources such as nuts, tofu and beans are so much better for your skin. And that's not just it because in your avocados and olive oil are present unsaturated fats that are healthy and provide fatty acids. These fatty acids keep the skin hydrated and the cell membranes strong so it's great if you cook your veggies in unsaturated oils such as olive oil, or flax oil and remember to use only a small amount!

So what is it that you're waiting for? A radiant skin awaits you, so stock up and fruits, vegetables, whole grains, beans and nuts and gives up the meat and dairy food. You will end up with a skin that shines with a genuine glow from the inside!

LONGER LIFE

Many studies have demonstrated that individuals that follow a vegan diet or follow a vegan/vegetarian lifestyle tend to live three to six years longer than those who don't.

You'll be surprised to know that just by switching from your average standardized diet to a vegan diet you can actually increase your life by thirteen years i.e. add thirteen more healthy years to your life. This has been claimed by Michael F. Roizen, MD, who is the author of The Real Age Diet: Make Yourself Younger with What You Eat. Consumption of saturated, four-legged fat results in the reduction of your life span and leaves you more disable as you grow towards the end of your life. This is because saturated unhealthy fat from animal products has the ability to clog your arteries as we have discussed that considerably slows down your immune system and drains your energy. Another matter of concern that arises from meat eating is that these consumers also end up with sexual dysfunction at a younger age and experience early cognitive deterioration.

To prove with an example let it be known to you that the people living in Okinawa, Japan have the longest life expectancy in the whole world and this has been proven by a study of more than 600 Okinawa centenarians over a period of 30 years. The interesting thing is that these Japanese people have a low calorie diet containing unrefined complex carbohydrates, soy, fruits and vegetables. This means they are vegans and experience longer lives more than almost all other populations of the world.

HAIR

As people have reported changed in their skin, they have also reported of improvements in their hair after they started on vegan diets. They say that their hair became stronger and has a lot more body and volume. Thanks to vegan diet, their hair looks a lot healthier now.

NAILS

Apart from hair and skin, healthy vegan diets have also shown beneficial results in nails making them stronger and healthier. Apparently, healthy nails are indicative of better overall health as well. So healthy nails is definitely good news.

BAD BREATH

Vegans have also noticed that since they switched to vegan diets they seem to have fresher breath in the morning. Sometimes, they can't even seem to remember the last their breath smelled bad. This is an obvious result of the type of food you eat. Due to vegan food, many vegans frequently experience a significant reduction in bad breath and wake up in the morning without having morning breath.

MIGRAINES

Another interesting advantage of vegan diet has been discovered. Individuals that suffer from migraine have also reported that when they go on vegan diets they often discover a great relief from their migraines.

BODY ODOR

It's true that whatever you eat is also expelled in your sweat and comes off as body odor. Thus, the elimination of dairy products and red meat from your diet means reducing body odor significantly. If you wish to smell better, just go vegan!

ALLERGIES

Apparently, there is an association of vegan diets to allergy symptoms as well. Reduced intake of meat, eggs and dairy eliminates allergy symptoms and it has been reported by many vegans that they experience much fewer congestion and runny nose problems.

PMS AND MENOPAUSE

PMS is a huge problem for several women out there and it appears that the elimination of dairy from your diet helps these women. Many women have said that after going vegan, PMS symptoms have considerably reduced, become a lot less intense and in some cases have even disappeared.

In addition to relieving you from PMS related symptoms, vegan diet will also ease the symptoms of menopause. There are many foods that have nutrients benefitting for the menopausal and premenopausal women. Some foods contain a rich amount of phytoestrogens that acts like estrogen and mimics its function. It is the plant-based chemical compound of estrogen. So if you maintain a good balance of phytoestrogens in your diet, you can pass through menopause without much trouble because they increase and decrease the levels of progesterone and estrogen favorably. What wouldn't women do to pass through menopause comfortably right? So this is a simple solution for those women out there. The greatest and primary source for phytoestrogens is soy but you can also find these compounds in other natural food sources including dates, apples, olives, cherries, yams, plums, garlic, squash and raspberries. Moreover, since menopause also causes weight gain and slows down your metabolism, a high-fiber and low-fat vegan diet is the best sort of diet for menopausal women and will help them shed any extra pounds they might gain.

OTHER BENEFITS

REDUCED POLLUTION

Many people become vegetarians not for the sole purpose of improving their own health but because they realize the devastating affects that the meat industry has on the environment. So by switching to a vegan lifestyle, you can help improve the environmental conditions by reducing pollution and preventing global climatic changes. Confined and crowded animal facilities and factory farms where animals are raised for the production of food are a huge cause of air, water and land pollution. Going on a vegan diet will be your contribution in helping Mother Earth become healthier and happier.

NO TOXIC CHEMICALS FOR YOU

It is estimated by the EPA that fish, meat and dairy products contain 95% of the pesticide residue in the typical American diet. By avoiding these food products you are saving yourself from ingesting pesticides. Meat and dairy products may be filled in with steroids and hormones that can be really bad for your health and fish in particular contain heavy metals.

HELP REDUCE FAMINE

Statistically, 70% of all the grain that is produced in the United States is fed to animals that are raised for slaughter. Also, the American population consumes five times less grain than the 7 billion livestock animals of the United States. This means that if all the grain that is consumed by the livestock was fed to the people instead, than you can feed nearly 800 million people with it and if it was exported than the US trade balance would rise by $80 billion a year.

SAVING ANIMALS AND PROTECTING THEIR RIGHTS

There are several vegans that give up their meat only because they are concerned about the animals and are against their suffering. These animals are not farmed freely on grounds, but in fact most of them are factory famed. In factory farms, animals are stuffed into cages that overcrowded. They can hardly move or even turn around. They are also fed a diet filled with antibiotics, hormones and pesticides and they spend their lives in crates. There are no laws for the protection of these farmed animals and are in fact specifically excluded from the state anticruelty laws for basic humane protection. Every year, ten billion animals are slaughtered for human consumption.

YOU WILL SAVE MONEY

For an average American, meat is 10% of his food spending. So if the 200 pounds of beef, fish and chicken that a meat eater has in a year is replaced with eating grains, fruits and vegetables then you would actually save an average of $4000 in a year.

A DINNER PLATE FULL OF COLORS

Fruits and vegetables contain disease-fighting phytochemical. These phytochemicals give these fruits and veggies their rich and different colors and hues. There are mainly two classes: carotenoids and anthocyanins. Carotenoids give all the rich yellow and orange vegetables and fruits such as mangoes, carrots, pumpkins, oranges, corn and sweet potatoes their color. On the other hand, the leafy greens are also rich in carotenoids but get their color from chlorophyll. Then fruits and vegetables containing anthocyanins are red, purple and blue such as cherries, plums and red bell peppers. So when you cook by color, you get to make sure that you're eating all the variety of natural substances, that are disease-fighting and that immunity boosting helping to prevent a range of illnesses.

CHAPTER 8 – SUCCESS STORIES

So you've taken a good look at the countless benefits that the vegan lifestyle brings with it but I am sure you still question the authenticity, and whether everything that has been stated about its advantages are true or not. Well, to remove any doubts that are running through your head, you'll find in this chapter a whole bunch of success stories from people that have truly experienced a great deal of positive changes in their lives with the help of the vegan diet and lifestyle.

Adopting veganism may be a little hard at first but it's completely worth it. Many people have shared their stories of how vegan diet and choosing a vegan lifestyle changed their life entirely and brought them health and happiness they have never had before. All over the world vegan diet has proved successful in reversing and preventing several diseases, improving unhealthy conditions and helping people shed several pounds. Who doesn't want that for themselves?

So take a look at some success stories and make them part of your motivation. These stories are reasons for you to take up the vegan diet and give up the meat!

So this young man thought that he was destined to live a life of obesity that would lead him towards nothing but misery and an early death. Since the age of sixteen, this young man, Jake Stevanga tried to get rid of his obesity and change this path of misery that he was following but unfortunately all in vain. In fact, he even tried playing several sports in the attempt to achieve weight loss and keep his body weight maintained but he realized that none of it was working and he wasn't just constantly obese but in fact, growing in size with every passing year. Sadly, nothing seemed to work and he felt that he lacked the knowledge that was needed to make a positive change so by the start of his twenties he had started losing hope, thinking obesity was his life-long partner. From that point onwards, it started getting really bad; it would take him an hour just to walk two miles.

Then, in 2013, he ran into a film called "Forks over Knives" which marked the turning point of his life. It was his life jacket, a life-saving miracle that turned everything around. From here, he got the information that he really needed to be able to live the life that he always wanted and knew he deserved. Inspired, he finally knew what to do! And from that day onwards, he lost 30 kilos of weight which is equivalent to 66 pounds and even ran the Melbourne Marathon without training for it.

SO THE QUESTION IS: HOW DID HE GET SO FAR SO QUICKLY?

One day after watching Forks over Knives, Jake came across the FOK Instagram that had posted about a plant-based, ultra-athlete Rich Roll. In that second, another epiphany struck: We are not bound to return our bodies to their natural state but we can actually take our body's health and performance to another level and achieve even more than average. He realized that it was possible to break paradigms of what he thought was possible and that blew his mind. So then, suddenly he decided that he was not just going to lose his excess fat and weight but he will expand his vision and aim for even better. He decided that to achieve this goal, he will go as far as it takes and will not give up. At the end of the day, it is all about determination that he had!

After losing 66 pounds/30 kilos in about four to five months, he stopped looking at the scale. After March 2014, he stopped stressing and worrying about his diet restrictions and his weight in general. He just focused on eating healthy, plant-base, and fresh foods. He just made sure he took care of himself and had food in the most natural and whole form that he could. And then the magic just started to happen on its own.

Jake used to tell his friends in early 2014 that he wished to run a marathon one day but at that time he wasn't able to run consistently for more than a mile. Judging his dream and situation, he put the idea of the marathon on the back burner and for the next six months, he decided on two goals: to train from the start in every session as hard as he could and to never ever give up. This was the best goal he ever set for himself.

After constant training for six months, one Sunday morning he woke up early and decided to take a run to a distant location in his city. So he set off. He felt unbelievable and with every step that he took, he felt himself getting faster and stronger. So he didn't think much and just ran, ran as much as he could and when he finally got to his destination, it struck him that he had successfully ran over 8.5 miles/14K! He had never in his life made that long a run before and he had broken his previous record, 3 miles, by a huge margin. According to him, the feeling of achievement was so immense and so wonderful that he was positively reinforced to run even more. So he actually ended up running over 12 miles/20K which half the distance in a marathon.

Even then he still didn't think much of running the marathon and thought that instead he'll give the half marathon a try but it was already sold out so he ended up signing up for the full marathon in Melbourne. Just his luck!

Through the entire course of the run Jakes main goal was to make sure that his heart, blood and other organs remained cool and healthy because he had never run that distance before and he didn't want to wind up causing any damage to his body that would stop him from ever running again. So he kept cautious and maintained his electrolytes throughout the race. He hit every water station and kept his hat wet as well. Only after 28 kilometers of running, he took a bite of his plant-based energy bar – one quarter at a time through the last 10 kilometers. To his surprise, and I am sure to yours as well he actually managed to complete the marathon in 4 hours and 50 minutes. He says that this was the most amazing and fun experience of his whole life!

So when you look at men like Jake, you realize how far they actually came with a positive switch in their life that completely turned it around. From being sick, miserable and obese, to watching Forks over Knives and then eventually successfully completing a marathon is extremely inspirational. It's truly amazing how eating plants can change one's life so drastically and so positively!

ANOTHER WOMAN LAURIE M FROM NORMAN, OK SHARES HER SUCCESS STORY

She claims that when she and her husband decided to go vegan, they virtually eliminated all chances of ever having heart or vascular diseases which were common and prevalent in their family. Their lipid profile indicates that they will probably never in their life need the quadruple coronary bypass surgeries that both of their fathers had to go through. She not maintains her weight at 110 pounds with the help of vegan diet that she now absolutely loves and can live with happily forever.

Kathy E, from Scottsdale, AZ

Around a year ago she was on Lipitor. She was overweight by about 25 pounds and had a cholesterol level of 234. Not only was she over weight but she had started showing early signs of arthritis in her fingers and was even on nasal and allergy medications. Then she took the smart decision of adopting a vegan diet and things turned around. Her cholesterol level dropped to 160, her allergies disappeared, the arthritis could no longer be found and she managed to lose over 25 pounds from her body. She no longer had to take any medications or depend on them for anything. Now, she feels a lot more energetic and always feels much better consistently. Her changes inspired her husband as well who also after opting for the vegan lifestyle lost 45 pounds and dropped his cholesterol level from 199 to 158.

ROBYN R FROM GLENDALE, AZ

Robyn and her family decided to eat vegan two years ago. According to her it was the most positive change that they adopted. Her husband lost 40 pounds of his weight in five months and even stopped taking Lipitor because the cholesterol level also dropped by 100 points. Surprisingly, this guy even improved his eye sight considerably that he had to get new contact lenses. Robyn herself lost 65 pounds over seven months and she says that she feels great! She feels that she has increased energy and healthy hair and nails but those are just the results that are visible to us but there are so many benefits that are inside our bodies and we can't see. If there is so much improvement on the outside, then the inside must be even better. Vegan diet has led her down a road to a healthy life. She is freed from diseases and has inspired her young boys of ages 6 and 9 to understand that importance of what we eat and how it makes a huge difference.

CHAPTER 9 – THE MEAT INDUSTRY

It's necessary that some light be shed on the meat industry in the United States and how it's lobbying the government to suppress public knowledge and keep secrets from the general public. Not many people know that the meat industry of the United States also acts as a huge and powerful political force that without spending large amounts of money targets a small number of regulators and key lawmakers. These lawmakers have a direct influence and impact on their business. So by exploiting these lawmakers, the meat industry has successfully prevented many meat-safety initiatives particularly in the recent years for the purpose of their own business success.

In America, the meat consumption is 8 ounces in a day which is twice the global average and in a year, 10 billion animals are slaughtered. Animal factories such as the Confined animal Feeding Operations (CAFO) use a lot of energy create pollution and cause a whole lot of environmental damage as well.

THE MEAT PRODUCERS

Meat trade and lobbying organizations represent many companies of the meat business and big meatpackers. These organizations include: The National Meat Association, the American Meat Institute and the National Cattlemen's Beef Association. Together, they are a powerful group and have a strong influence on the government. They make sure that whenever bills are enacted, or regulations are finalized, they are part of the decision making process and influence any decisions, especially those affecting meat business.

There are four companies in the United States that produce 85% of all the beef in the United States:

- Tyson Foods (TSN)
- JBS (JBSAY)
- Cargill
- Smithfield Foods

TYSON FOODS (TSN)

Tyson Foods bought Iowa Beef Processors in 2001 and became the world's largest poultry and red meat provider. Today, it has control over 27% of all the meat and poultry that is sold in the United States, which means that 1 out of every 4 pounds of beef, chicken or pork consumed in the United States is a Tyson product. Tyson has 59 plants with 50,000 employees which easily makes it the largest poultry processing company in the U.S. Tyson supplies many restaurant chains across the country including Kentucky Fried Chicken and McDonalds. Kettle Cooked Foods, Russer, Lady Aster, Jordan's, Tasty bird, Iowa Ham, Nature's Farm organic chicken, Weaver and ITC are brands under the Tyson parent company.

SLAUGHTER HOUSES

"Knockers" which are slaughterhouse workers drive steel bolts into the heads of cows to stun them while others hang them by their hooves with the help of chains and slit their jugular veins. The law requires that the animal must bleed to death before it is sent forward to the disassembly line to be skinned and dissected but that's not the case at Tyson slaughterhouse in Wallula, Washington. A worker from there has reported that cattle are processed so fast that they are still half conscious during the procedure. In fact, an affidavit states that "10% to 30% of animals at the IBP plant proceed through the skinning and dismemberment process in a fully conscious state." The conditions at the slaughterhouse are ruthless and cruel; many workers have lost fingers and teeth, have had grave stab wounds, and have been attacked and kicked by animals gone wild. The workers themselves have even recorded animals on camera that were struggling while being skinned alive as they hung down chains.

This is not it. The torture to animals is endless. Birds like turkeys, chicken, geese and ducks are not protected from any cruelty by laws regarding farm animals and that include humane slaughter. Completely conscious and alive turkeys and chickens are hung by their upside-down by their ankles to a moving conveyer belt. Then in order to immobilize them, the birds are given intense and agonizing electric shocks so that it becomes easier to slit them by their throats. The shocks don't necessarily work every time and the chickens remain conscious. Once that is done, they are slashed along their throats using a mechanical blade but sometime, some of them escape the blade and are moved on to the scalding tank station still alive and breathing. At these stations, birds are drowned in scalding hot water, around 143 degrees F, contained in large tanks. The United States Department of Agriculture has reported that millions of birds in a year, which are submerged in scalding hot water, are fully conscious. A former worker at the Tyson slaughterhouse is reported to have claimed that at this point the conscious chickens are so devastated that they scream, kick, flop and struggle. They fight it so much that when they come of the other end of the tank, they are disfigured and even have broken bones.

KENTUCKY FRIED CHICKEN & MCDONALDS

The PETA sponsored a campaign called the "Kentucky Fried Cruelty" to create pressure on KFC and force it to give up Tyson Foods as its primary meat supplier because of its cruel and abusive behavior towards animals and because of its resistance to improve methods.

Interestingly, back in May 2005, two animal welfare experts refused to sign an agreement that excluded them from speaking openly regarding the issue of animal slaughter; they resigned from their positions. Moreover, when Dr. Temple Grandin and Dr. Ian Duncan were asked to sign an agreement that required them to discuss all media inquiries with KFC corporate headquarters, they also gave up their place in the YUM! Brands (the parent company of KFC) animal welfare committee and stepped down.

Not only has PETA campaigned against KFC but they have long been campaigning against McDonald's as well. McDonald's seriously lacks any animal welfare standards and they even violate the most minimal of government standards as well. For two years, PETA discussed the McDonalds issue and tried to convince them but when all was in vain they finally launched the McCruelty to go campaign against McDonalds in 1999.

100% cows are supposed to be completely stunned before they are skinned as required by the Federal standards however, the McDonald's training video says that 5 conscious cows in every 100 while being skinned and dissected is acceptable.

SMITHFIELD FOODS

Then there is Smithfield Foods, which is the world's greatest pork producer. In the United States, Smithfield has the largest pig farming operation and is also a major producer outside of the country. 26% of the U.S. pork market is under the control of Smithfield that is raising 14 million pigs and killing 27 million out of the 60 million that made it to the slaughter house back in 2006. Recently, the company has started beef operations as well and is the fifth largest beef packer. Smithfield Foods is also leading in the production of processed foods and deli meat.

The company has expanded many operations and exports abroad as well and has made over 20 acquisitions since 1981 when it was only producing pork regionally. Smithfield's success and growth has remained unobstructed by any anti-trust actions and without any protest or resistance from the U.S. Department of Agriculture (USDA), the 2003 acquisition of the bankrupt Farmland Foods elevated the company from 20-27% of the market. Moreover, in spite of hog waste run-offs that horribly polluted the rivers and turned them into toxic dumps, the Environmental Protection Agency (EPA) campaign against immense water pollution that came from its Virginia and North Carolina factories was not taken very seriously. Smithfield foods also very comfortably rejected and denied any state laws that prohibited meat packers from owning the animals that they slaughtered. Smithfield has been a great source of animal cruelty and environmental damage. What it has successfully achieved in these aspects is something you should know:

In the Smithfield warehouses, the hogs live by the hundreds or thousands and are arranged in rows of wall-to-wall pens. They are so overly crowded and cramped inside that the cages appear too small for them to even move in. The sows are impregnated artificially, and are made to deliver their piglets in these crammed conditions and cages that are almost so tiny that they can't even turn around. And then are huge 250 pound male hogs, around 40 in number that are made to live in a pen the size of a small apartment. They are so incredibly crowded in there that they often trample each other to death because they literally have no space. These animals are completely deprived of any fresh air, sunlight or even straw and land. Their excrement is allowed to fall into pits underneath as the floors are slated. But these pits unfortunately don't contain excrement only because almost anything can end up in them including broken insecticide bottles, antibiotic syringes, or even piglets that are still-born or accidentally crushed by their mothers.

There are foot-wide pipes that drain these pits and remain closed until there is enough waste and sewage gathered in the pits to create sufficient expulsion pressure. Then the pipes are allowed to open up and expel everything they contain into a large pound. So everything the pits contain bursts out of the pipes and winds up in these ponds. Moreover, sometimes the temperatures in these warehouses rise tremendously and go above 90 degrees and the air is filled with chemicals, dust and excrement that in order to keep it clean a huge exhaust fan must be running all day and night long. Because if the exhausts don't work for even the smallest amount of time, the pigs start dying due to the contaminated air that is impossible to breathe in.

After Tyson Foods, the second largest meat producer of the U.S. is Cargill. It is also the second largest animal feed supplier in the world.

It is said these companies hold a lot of power over what goes on and they exploit their influence to depress the farmers pay while keeping the prices for consumers much higher! It is because of these companies that the price of meat keeps becoming higher but the quality continues to decline and this is kept from the general public. They are not warned that their health is at stake.

There are many examples in history that have been quoted and provide evidence of the evil-doings of the meat industry. For example, in 1995, the Meat industry used its power to prevent food-safety regulations. This happened after the Jack in the Box E.coli outbreak that devastatingly had 700 people sick. As a result the USDA proposed the formation and implementation of new food-safety laws. This was when the meat industry made attempts to delay and prevent the implementation of the new regulations by getting a member of the key appropriations committee on their side and convinced him to introduce an amendment to end the rulemaking process.

Another time in 1996, James Walsh, an upstate New York Republican proposed an amendment that forced the USDA to carry out detailed hearings which delayed the implementation of food-safety system. He had received over $65,000 from agriculture industry interests in the 1996 election cycle. The food-safety system that got delayed included a test for the presence salmonella in ground beef. The meat industry expressed objections towards the new salmonella testing by claiming that it was an improper scientific measure. They convinced James Walsh and made him offer the amendment on the industry's behalf.

WHAT THE MEAT INDUSTRY DOESN'T WANT YOU TO KNOW!

We rely on our meat industries blindly, and consider that as long as our meat looks clean, it's fine. But we have been unaware and kept under shadows by the meat industry. We don't know how they produce their meat, how they manufacture it, what they do to the animals and how they are kept. As we know, that the meat industry uses money and political power to lobby the government and suppress public knowledge of what the public deserves to know, let us look into some of those things that the meat industry has been hiding and paying lawmakers and regulators to shove underneath the carpet.

FOOD BOURNE DISEASES

Methods used in slaughterhouses and factory farms are not necessarily the healthiest. The methods used induce a risk of food borne illnesses in almost all the meat and dairy products, and eggs in the United States. Unfortunately, as of now there are no tests taken for food borne diseases and there is no such requirement thanks to the lobbying successfully done by the meat and dairy industries. The conditions of slaughterhouses are insane where cows are kept and raised in large fields that are almost the size of cities. Obviously, in such a huge cow population there is no check and the cows are smeared with fecal matter and filth. There are no actions taken to improve these conditions. The slaughterers are also kept under a lot of pressure with a lot of workload, as they are often made to kill and gut around 300 animals only in one hour.

Studies prove statistics that in around 50% (which is half!!) of the cattle carcasses, you can find the E.coli bacteria and it has also been estimated that approximately 70% of the chicken, and 90% of the Turkey found in stores contains harmful bacteria as well.

The primary source of Campylobacter, which is the leading bacteria in causing food-borne diseases and illnesses, is contaminated chicken flesh. A single chicken warehouse alone contains around 50,000 birds that are not closely taken care of. Additionally, the use of antibiotics makes them more susceptible to bacterial diseases as the bacteria continue to develop resistance against them. It has been reported that in the United States, approximately 5000 people in a single day contract food poisoning thanks to Campylobacter. Apart from Campylobacter, in the U.S., Salmonella is also frequently discovered infecting the chickens people consume. This, however, is not the case in Europe where animal treatment is better, more humane and animals are given more space. As a result, they do not fall victim to as many pathogens and suffer from diseases related to them. In fact, the Centers for Disease Control has even confirmed that there are Salmonella outbreaks from almost all animal products, such as pork, beef, egg and dairy.

This sad state of meat industry that everyone continues to conveniently ignore is a big reality that needs to be addressed. This is one of the reasons, including how animals are treated in these animal factories and slaughterhouses, for choosing veganism as a lifestyle. The worse bit is that instead of correcting the factory farm conditions and fixing the same, the U.S. meat industry makes use of nuclear radiation and irradiation to get rid of the pathogenic bacteria.

HORMONES AND ANTIBIOTICS

Before animals are slaughtered and used as food, they are treated with hormones or antibiotics. In the United States, above 90% of the beef cattle is fed hormones and in bigger cattle lots, the statistics even suggested 1000%. Recombinant bovine growth hormone (rbGh) is a genetically engineered hormone made by Monsanto that artificially induces an increase in the milk production of cattle by 10-15%. The use of rbGh was approved by the Food and Drug Administration (FDA) but it was declined in Europe and Canada both because apparently, cows that are injected with rbGh are said to have a 50% increase in lameness and 25% increase in udder infections.

Another hormone that is given to cows is the Growth Factor 1, created by Posilac. This growth hormone is the same in humans and cows both which is why it is considered as a reason for cancer growth and has been recognized in rapidly growing cancer. The problem is not just the harmful cancer induction or diseases, but also that cows find it difficult to adapt to high milk yields properly or even high grain diets. Additionally, infertility problems and metabolic disorders are also seen very commonly. The Consumers Union has stated that strong evidence exists in support of the health risks associated with rbGh.

Animals are not only treated with the hormones mentioned above but also with antibiotics. It would have made more sense if antibiotics were used only for the purpose of treating sick animals but surprisingly, U.S. livestock producers use 24.6 million pounds of antibiotics in a year for other non-therapeutic purposes. This means that as opposed to treating sick animals, a huge amount of antibiotics is used only for the purpose of enhancing growth and preventing diseases. That is an unjustified excessive use of antibiotics. Out of the 24.6 million used non-therapeutically, 10.5 million is used in poultry, 3.7 million on cattle and 10.3 million is used on hogs. In comparison, humans only use 3 million pounds of antibiotics annually in the United States. It has been reported that the antibiotics administered to animal is around eight times more than the amount used by people for diseases.

FEEDING WASTE PRODUCTS TO LIVESTOCK

It might come to you as a surprise that on top of the filthy conditions that the animals are already kept in, they are also fed with sewage sludge and dried poultry waste. Even though, in 1997 the FDA finally banned the feeding of cow meat and bone meal to cows, chickens and often pigs are given feathers, bones, brains, meat scraps, and their own feces routinely. This trash and waste material is part of the daily diet of animals that we consume as meat and dairy. Our eggs and meat come from animals that, on a daily basis, consumed cat and dog remains, and even had euthanasia drugs injected in them. Imagine that you actually eat livestock that was fed 40 billion pounds of slaughterhouse wastes such as blood, bone, viscera and even dead cats and dogs that were euthanized at the veterinarians and animal shelters. Unfortunately, but honestly that is a disgusting and repulsive way not only to treat animals but is also an evil act towards unaware humans.

DISEASES FROM FARMING

MAD COW DISEASE

The World Health Organization passed seven recommendations in response to young people in England dying of Creutzfeldt - Jakob disease which is the human equivalent of Mad cow disease, It must be highlighted, that the United States to this date continues to violate four of these concrete recommendations out of which the first one is to cease the feeding of animals to each other. A GAO report from 2002 claims that boiled skeletal remains of carcasses are used in beef extract and beef stock. And even more surprising is the fact that hamburgers, taco fillings, hot dogs and pizza toppings contain spinal cord contamination.

CHICKEN CANCER AND BIRD FLU

The United Nations claim that bird/avian flu is the result of over-crowded, filthy and disease ridden factory farm conditions that we have discussed. Evidence also supports that in some chicken farms; almost 90% of the chickens are infected with leukosis/chicken cancer.

PNEUMONIA AND SWINE FLU

In factory farms, there is production of toxic gases and irritating fumes. There is also dust and bacteria build up because of over-crowded warehouses. This causes factory pigs to develop respiratory distress and infections that are also caught by the workers. Statistics reveal that around 80% of the pigs in the Unites States have pneumonia when they are slaughtered and the water that is given to these pigs is usually the liquid waste from manure pits. This is the reason for the outbreaks of diseases such as swine flu!

CHAPTER 10 – ETHICAL VEGANISM – THE PHILOSOPHY

Ethical Veganism forms the basis of the entire philosophy. The concept lies on the fact that animals like humans have rights and we have a responsibility towards animals to protect them instead of using them for our personal benefits. Animals have desires, beliefs, memory and the ability to pursue goals which makes them possess value as "subjects-of-a-life."However the right of remaining unharmed can be dismissed by other moral principles but reasons like food, pleasure and convenience are not good enough.

Right theorists also argue that all beings have one right to them if not any other, which is the right not to be treated as property. And we do exactly the opposite to animals and treat them as though we own them and can do whatever we want with them. So they say that if you feel that animals have intrinsic moral value, then veganism should be your first choice without a doubt.

As discussed in the start, people choose veganism for different reasons which make their type different as well. How you choose to follow veganism obviously depends on your reason for opting in the first place. Some people that follow a vegan diet may also never use animal products for other reasons as well. For example, a vegan may not wear animal products not for ethical reasons but may be health reasons that products used on the skin enter the body, or another vegan may not wear an animal product because it has a certain effect on the environment.

So this shows how vegans fall into several kinds depending on their reasons and intentions for being vegan. Similarly, those adopt veganism for spiritual or ethical reasons also fall into different groups. It depends on what they want to achieve, or what they stand against or simply the statement they wish to make. Some ethical vegans see their vegan diet as a mean to reduce animal suffering. They don't necessarily think that using animal for food is wrong or even killing them is wrong but they just think that it is wrong to cause pain and suffering to animals. They think that if there was a painless way of raising and slaughtering animals, they would not object to using animals for eating or other purposes. So such people don't have a problem with the exploitation animals for their use. They just have concerns regarding the pain and suffering it causes.

Basically ethical veganism takes veganism beyond vegan diet and opposes animal consumption in any form. They pursue a vegan diet and do not wear animal products, they reject co modification of nonhumans as property and they also believe that animal based farming harms other humans and non-humans. They link human rights to animal rights and believe that there is not much difference between the two. They believe that animal exploitation should be completely abolished and so ethical veganism forms the moral baseline for the animal rights movement.

People that go vegan for ethical and not dietary reasons think that humans do not have the right to abuse or oppress animals and other species because they are not as intellectual. Human rights and animal rights go hand in hand for ethical vegans because both have the ability to feel pleasure, pain and fear and are capable of experiencing suffering as well.

Of all the veganism approaches, ethical veganism promises the most consistent behavior because vegans for health reasons may end up cheating just like people on other diets do. Or environmental vegans may weigh the adverse environmental consequences between an animal and non-animal product and decide against the animal product that may be it is less harmful. And people that think of veganism as a way of reducing suffering may be in a situation where they think that not using the animal product may actually cause more suffering and end up using it. However, a truly ethical vegan believes that veganism is an approach to life, with a strong philosophy of living behind it.

CHAPTER 11 – ENVIRONMENTAL VEGANISM

You have been given all information regarding the vegan diet, dietary vegans and the ethical vegans as well. Now let's take a look into the third kind of vegans called the environmental vegans. These vegans are focused on conservation. Animal rights are not their purpose for veganism.

Environmental vegans are against the use of animal products because they come from factory farming, hunting, fishing and trapping. They believe that these practices are environmentally unsustainable and to an extent damaging for the environment.

Animal agriculture and farming has been linked to environmental damage in a report by the United Nations Food and Agriculture Organization. The report stated that livestock farming of pigs, chicken and cows affected all parts of the environment: air, water, land, soil, climate and even biodiversity. Livestock farming is responsible for a great amount of air pollution because according to the report, it was responsible for 9% of carbon dioxide emissions, 65% of nitrous oxide, 37% of methane and 68% of ammonia.

Livestock waste accounts for the emission of 30 million tonnes of ammonia annually which induces the production of acid rain. This is why only by switching towards a vegan diet you can save the world from climate change, hunger and even fuel shortages.

AIR POLLUTION

Global warming is a result of the production of carbon dioxide, methane, and nitrous oxide. Did you know that the production of only 2 pounds of beef produces more greenhouse gases than driving a car for 3 hours? And it also takes up more energy than leaving your lights on in the house for three hours as well. The United Nations agree that in order to combat the global warming and climatic change, a global shift towards vegan diet is necessary! It has been estimated that livestock and their byproducts are responsible for at least 51% of the greenhouse gas emissions worldwide.

Apart from the greenhouse gases, factory farms also emit a great amount of dust and other contaminants that cause air pollution. Studies have provided evidence that animal feedlots in Texas contribute 7000 tons of dust to the air every year which contains mold, fungus, and bacteria from the feed and feces. Moreover, there are cesspools that contain tons of feces and urine. When they get full, factory farms spray liquid manure into the air which carried away by the wind and naturally, inhaled by the residents living nearby. Reports have even stated that animal wastes release toxic airborne chemicals that can lead to immune, inflammatory and neurochemical problems in humans that inhale these chemicals.

WATER POLLUTION

It's not that difficult to understand that factory farms obviously produce billions of pounds of manure which goes into rivers, lakes, streams and drinking water.

Factory farm animals produce one trillion pounds of waste that is used for the fertilization of crop. It is then subsequently run off into waterways, containing bacteria and other drugs. This water eventually goes and settles into giant pits in the ground or on crops resulting in the pollution of ground water and air both. In fact, the water run-off from agricultural sites is the main source of pollution in all waterways.

Excrement from factory farms is carried by rivers, streams and other running waters in to the Mississippi River which runs into the Gulf of Mexico thus depositing all its waste there. Nitrogen from fertilizers used to grow crops and from animal feces causes the growth of algae in water bodies. The algae take up all the oxygen in the water hardly leaving any behind for other life forms. This situation has resulted in the formation of "dead zone" at the Gulf of Mexico where almost all the sea animals and plants have died. According to a study by the Princeton University in 2006, if Americans were to shift from meat production and adopt vegan/vegetarian diets then the amount of nitrogen depositing in the gulf would be drastically reduced and the dead zone will become almost non-existent!

FACTS RELATING MEAT PRODUCTION TO ENVIRONMENTAL DAMAGE

- If a single person switches from meat eating to a vegan diet, they'll help to reduce carbon dioxide emission by 1.5 tons in a year
- If every American gave up only one serving of chicken in a week from their diet, they would save an amount Co2 emissions equal to taking 500,000 cars of the road.
- The largest producers of methane in the U.S. are chickens, pigs, cows and turkeys.
- 65% of the world's nitrous oxide emission is produced by the meat, egg and dairy industries
- A single calorie from animal protein needs eleven times more fossil fuel than one calorie of plant protein
- Meat eaters diets makes seven times more greenhouse gas emissions than vegan diets
- Half of all the water in the United States that is used is taken for the purpose of raising animals for food
- The production of only 1 pound of meat takes 2400 gallons of water whereas 1 pound of wheat only takes 25 gallons
- Surprisingly, you can actually save more water by no eating 1 pound of meat than you can save by not showering for six months
- A meat-eaters diet requires 4000 gallons of water in a day while a vegan diet only requires 300 gallons of water per day
- Around 89000 pounds of excrement per second is created from animals being raised for food. This makes a huge amount of groundwater pollution
- 35000 miles of rivers in 22 states have already been polluted with cattle, chicken and hog manure
- 30% of the earth's land mass is used for raising animals for food. That's almost the same size as Asia!
- Livestock grazing is the primary cause of extinction of plant species in the United States

The above mentioned facts easily convince you why certain people are so strongly against meat eating. Their concerns about the environment are absolutely genuine and the fact they do not eat meat actually makes a difference to Mother Earth. One can start by giving up one meal of meat in a day and then move ahead to give up more and you can create a huge difference. Being part of a simple process such as veganism to make the environment cleaner and healthier is doing a great service to the Earth, to you and to all other humans and non-humans that live in it!

Conclusion

This detailed book about veganism has finally come to an end and has you convinced why veganism is a great decision for you, your family and those around you. By making this life-changing decision you are not just going to make yourself happy, but you will also do Mother Earth, its water, its animals, and its air a huge favor. You will also make those around you happy and you may even end up inspiring people in the best and most positive of ways. You just have to take the first step and then promise to remain determined. So many people have done it, which means so can you.

By switching to a vegan diet you allow yourself to tread lightly on the planet and show compassion towards everything that lives on it. Now that you know about so many vegan recipes, you have a great number of vegan options! You never thought that eating green could be so delicious. So at the end of knowing everything about the vegan diet, its benefits, the environment and the meat industry, why you go vegan is your own choice. But remember that no matter what reason you choose for yourself, you have the power to bring a change into this world simply by bringing a change into what you have on your plate every day.

Before you opened this book you were asking why go vegetarian, and at the end of this book what you really should be asking is: Why haven't you gone vegetarian?